JACQUAY AND MR. SLEEP

Written by

Ella McCrea

Illustrated by

Sonia Morris

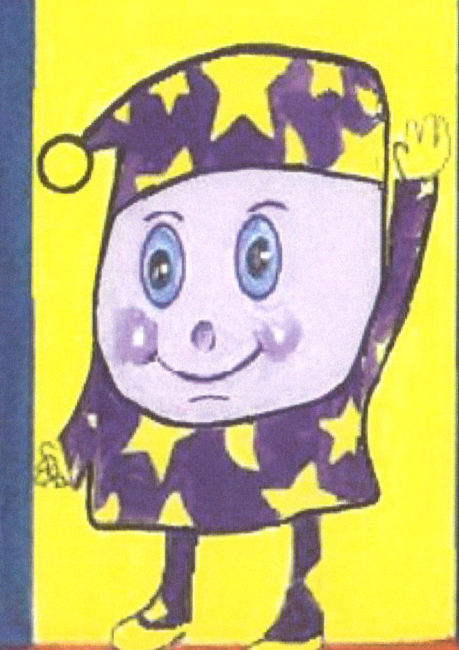

TOYS

ISBN: 978-1-63073-025-3

Available through the author and
Amazon and Barnes & Noble websites:
Amazon.com
BN.com

ACKNOWLEDGMENTS:

PINAWOR (Pinellas Authors and Writers Organization). Group meetings with PINAWOR have been a great encouragement and great writing support to me. I appreciate this organization and all its support.

Lenair Henriquez, Certified Leadership Coach and owner of Strategic Profile Solutions

Dorthia Patterson, Lanorus L. McCrea and Levette T. McCrea. Thanks for all your support in the creation of Jacquay and Mr. Sleep. I greatly appreciate all that you have done.

Special thanks to each of you!

FROM THE AUTHOR:

I have enjoyed writing this story for you to read. I hope you have lots of fun reading ***Jacquay and Mr. Sleep.***

Published by:

FL Publishers • North Fort Myers, FL 33903 • 888.720.0950

19 18 17 16 15 14   1 2 3 4 5

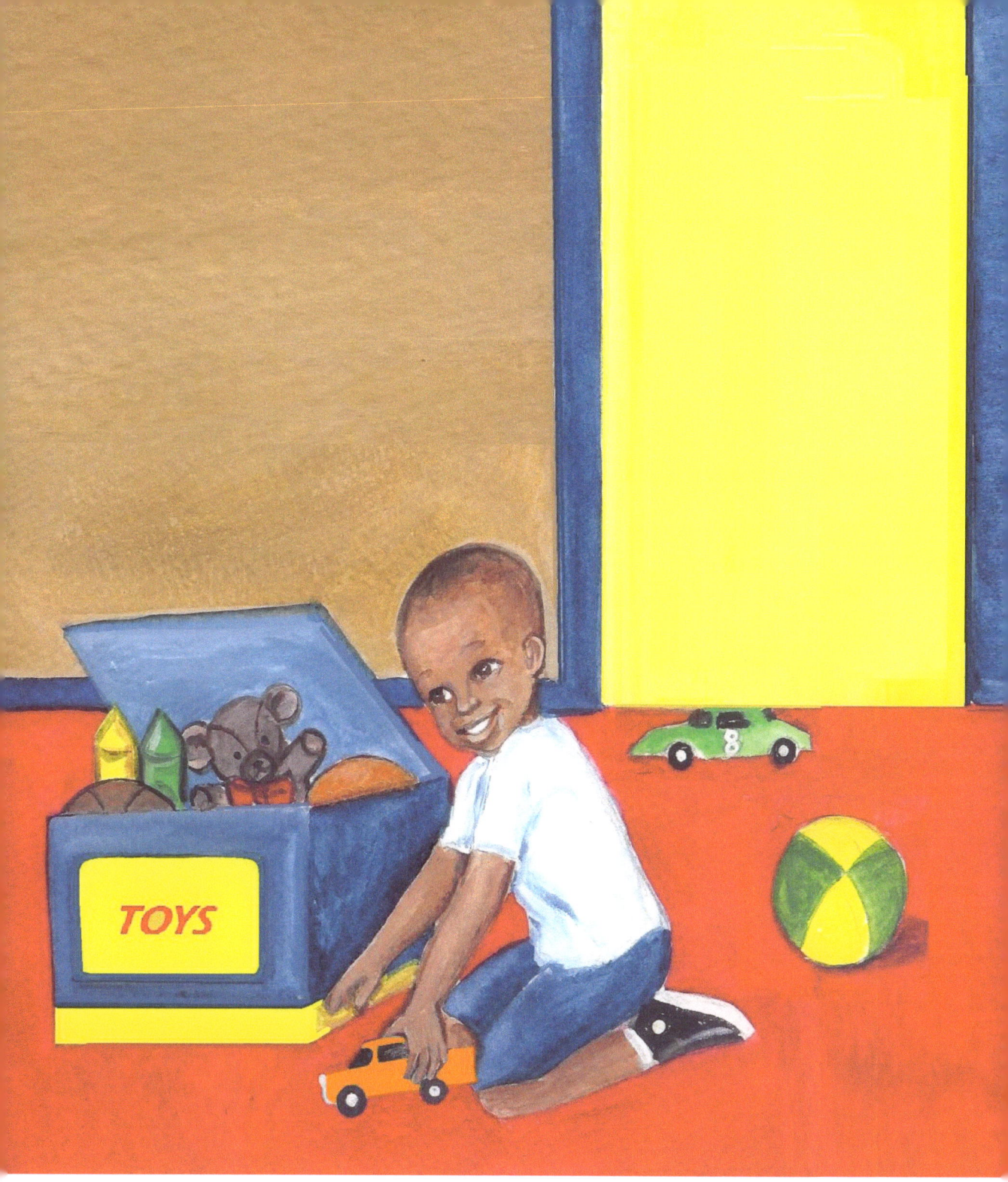

Jacquay was a little boy who loved to play. He
loved to play so much that he hated to go to sleep.

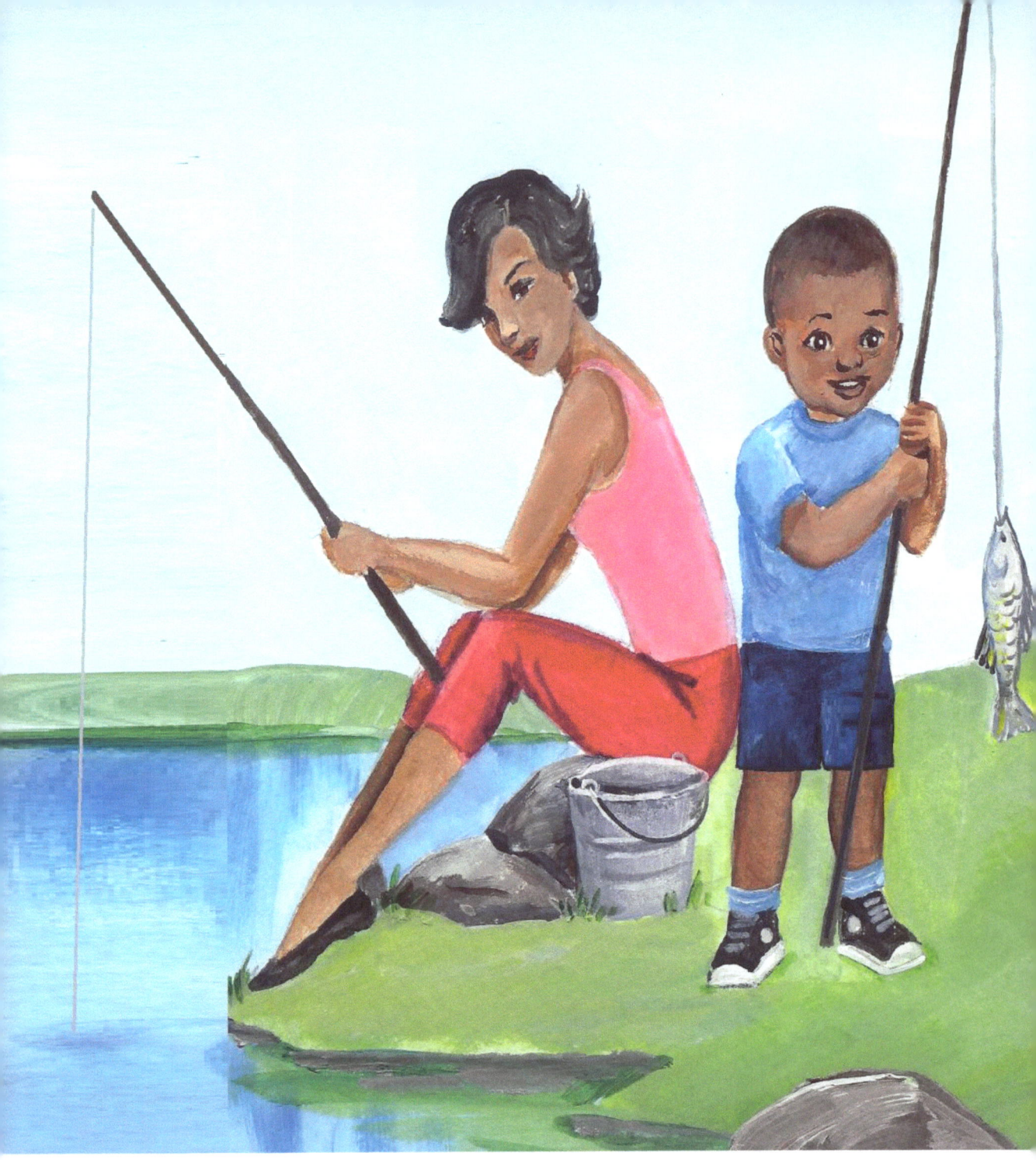

He had a wonderful mother who made sure
he had lots of fun things to do.

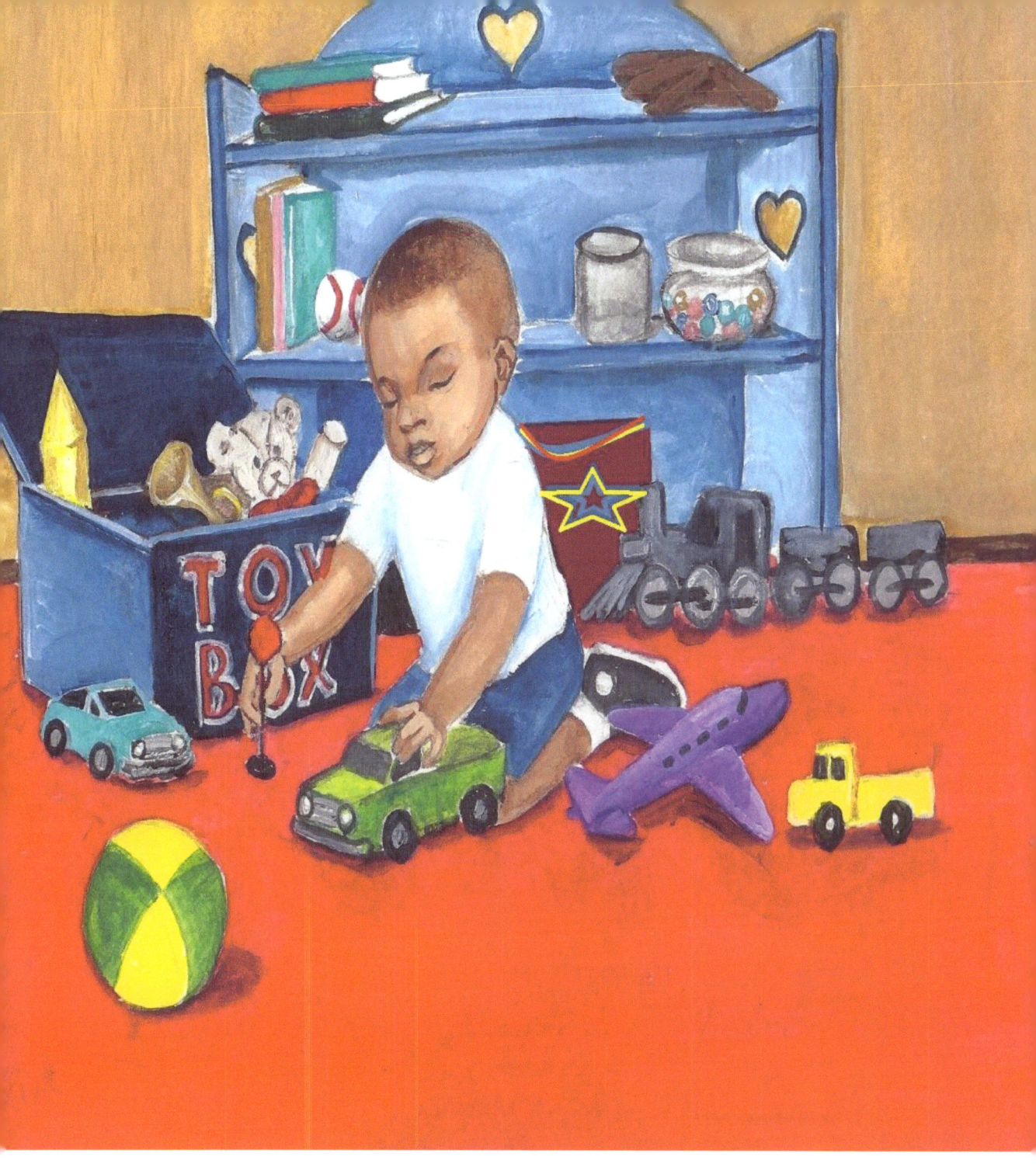

Jacquay had marbles in jars, tools, and toy cars.
He had airplanes, blocks, and trains.

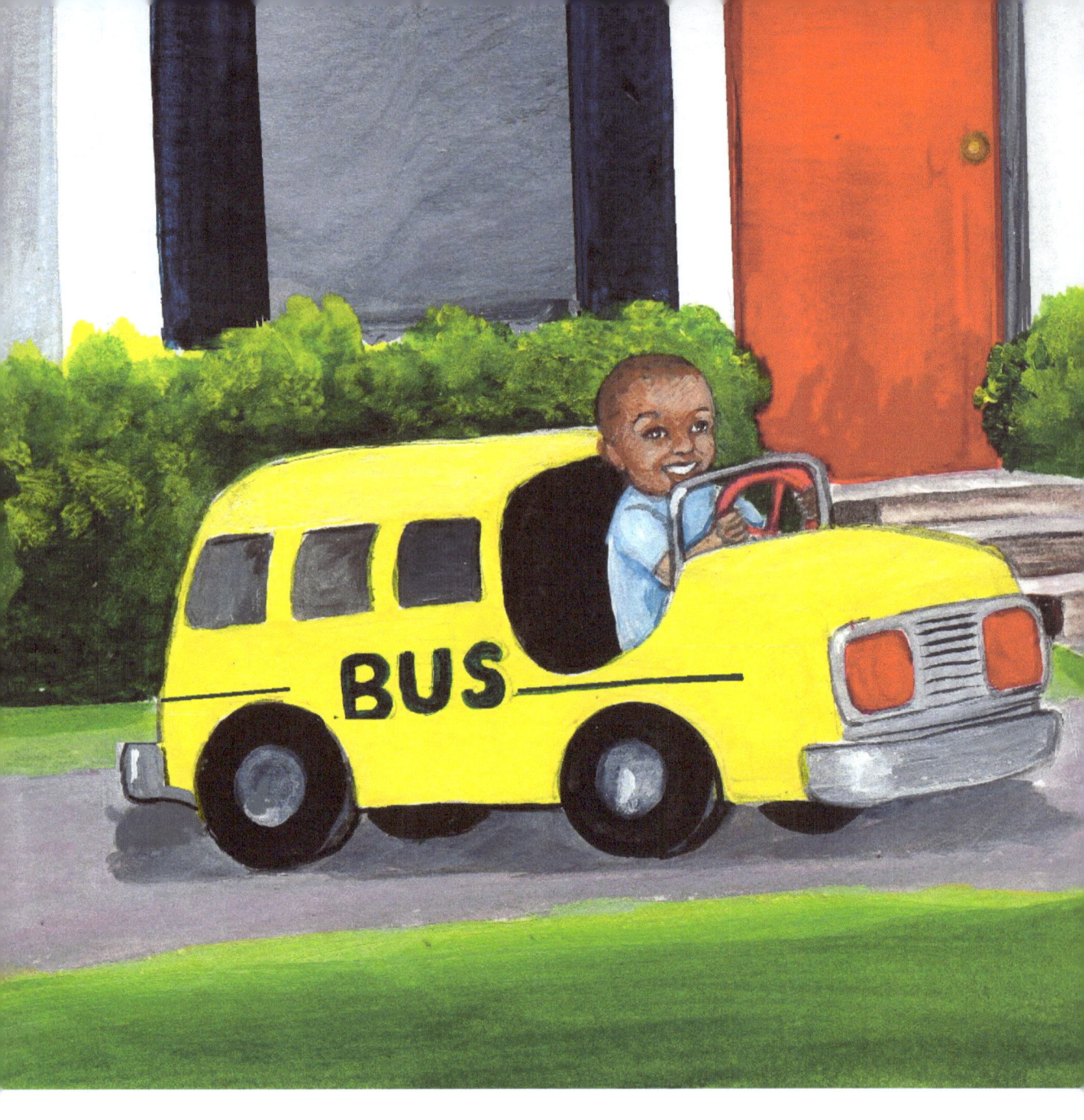

Jacquay had a bike and a radio with a mike.
He had a toy Santa, an elf, and a big yellow
bus that moved by itself.

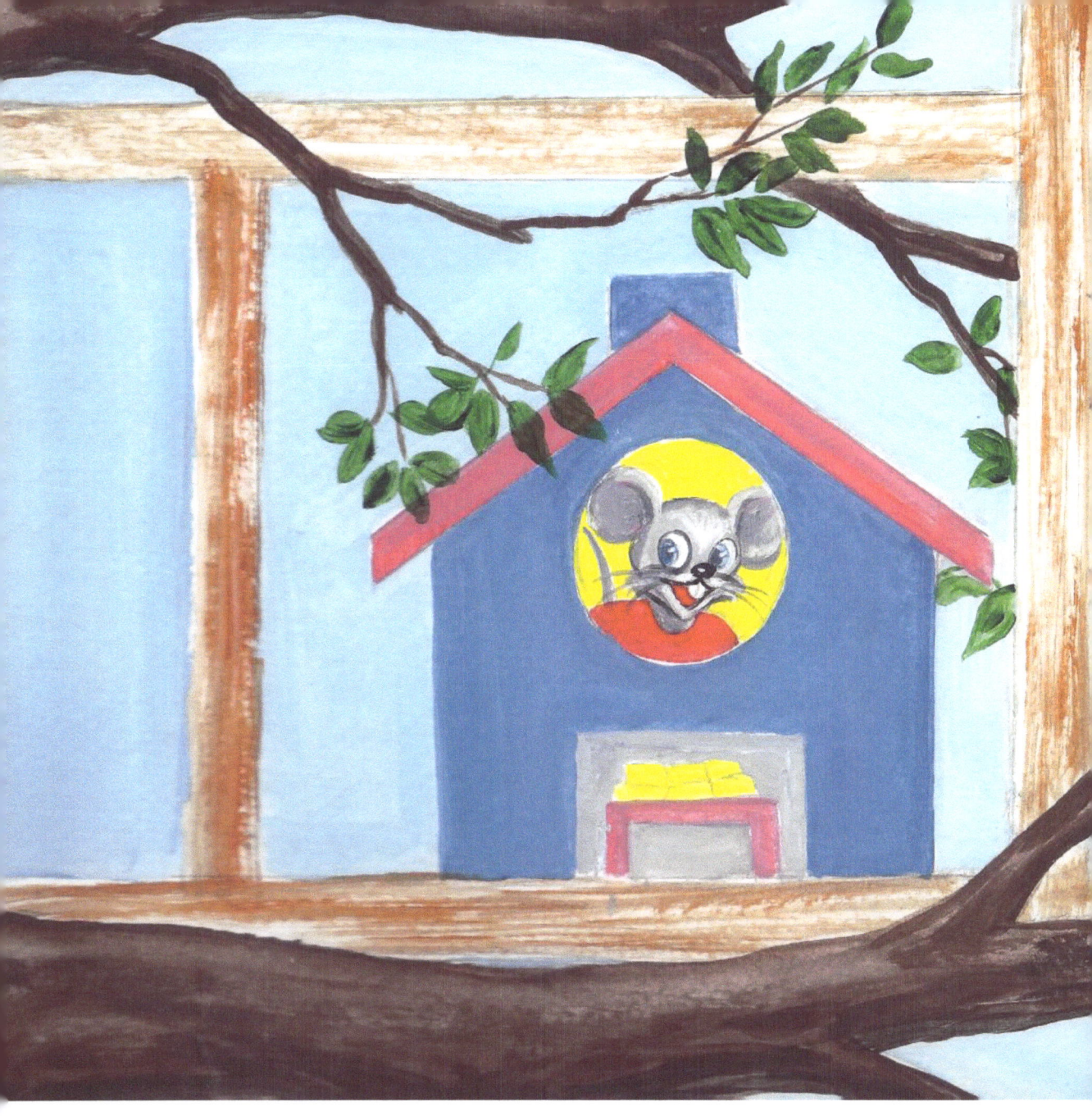

He had collections of rocks and leaves. He had a big playhouse in the trees. He had a beautiful little toy house for Adwin, his special pet mouse.

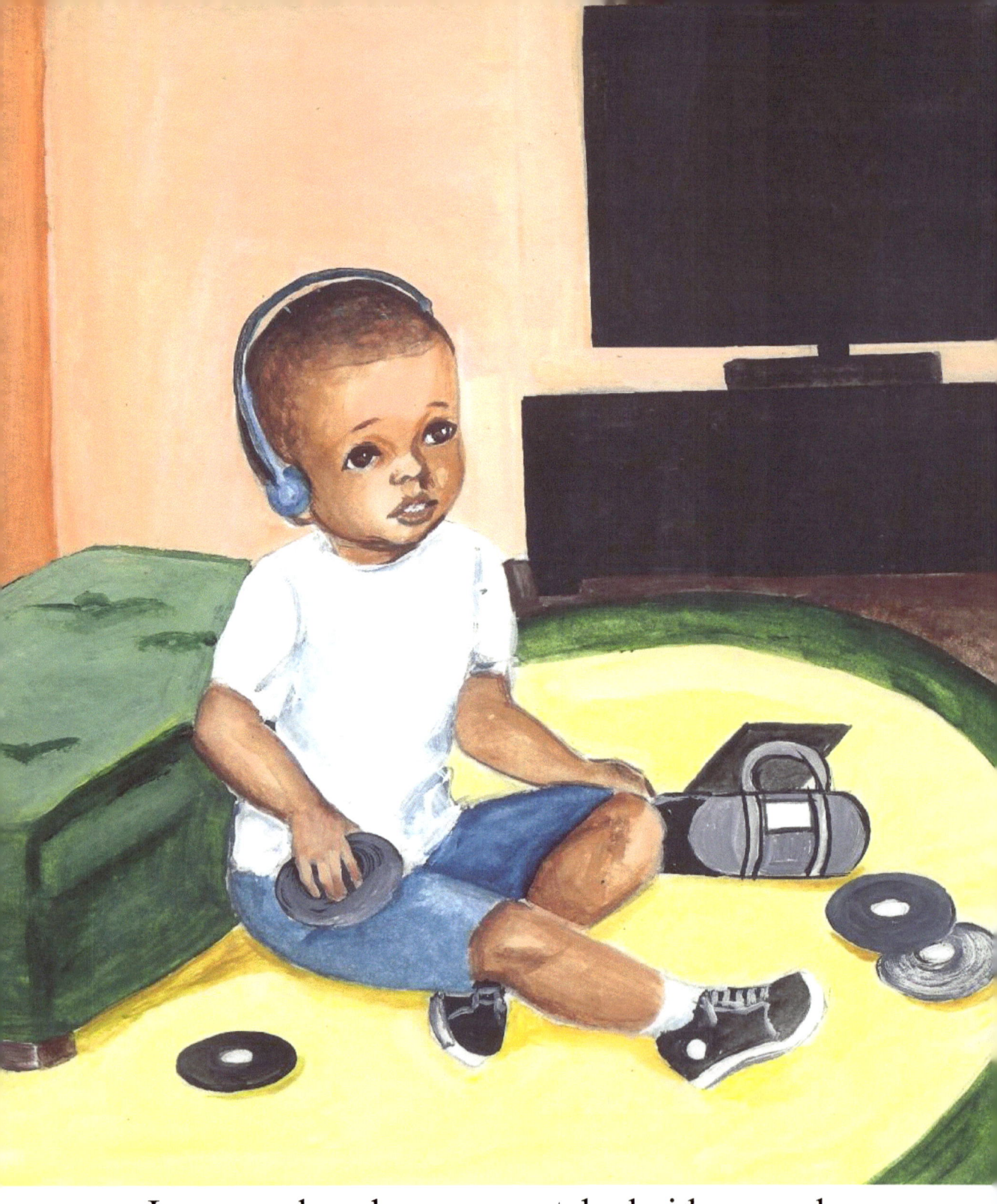

Jacquay played games, watched videos, and listened to music on his stereo.

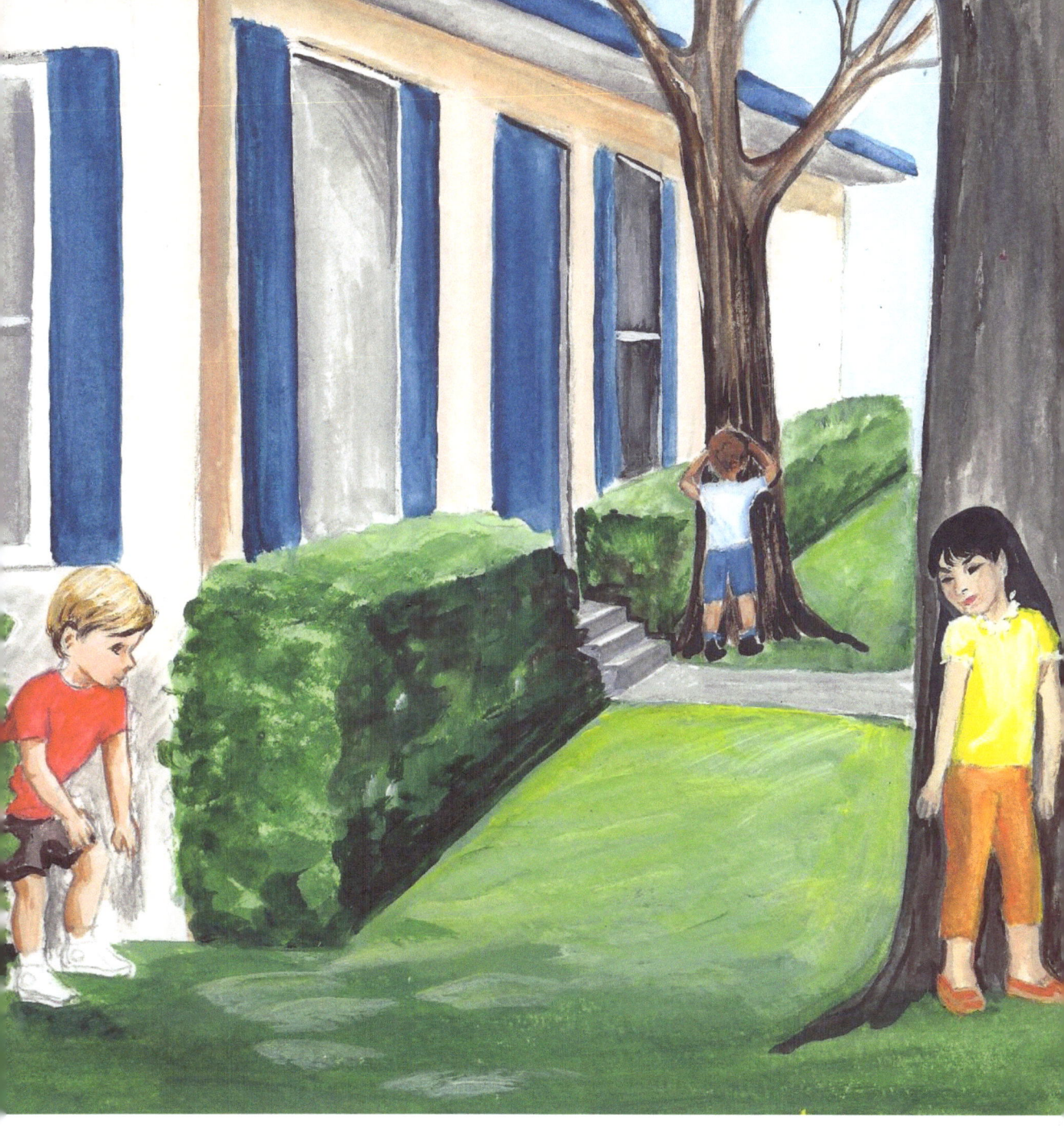

Sometimes Jacquay went over to play with Cindy and Pete, two friends who lived across the street. They played fun games like tag a winner and hide-n-seek.

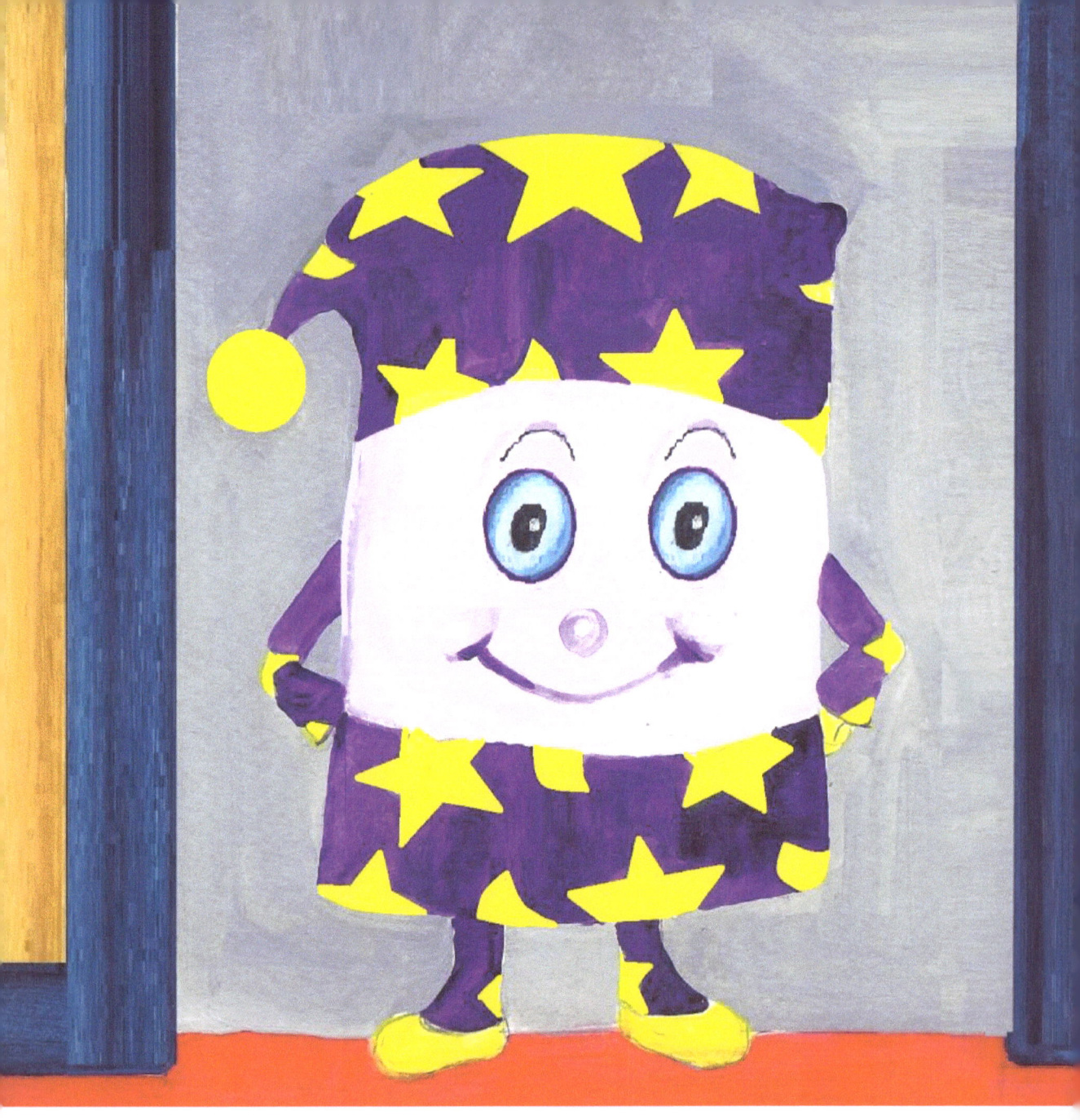

Jacquay loved his friends very much. But he had another friend that he knew nothing about. His name was Mr. Sleep. Mr. Sleep came around every day, always more than once. He never came before breakfast, but always after lunch. Mr. Sleep was calm and very quiet. Sometimes he tiptoed when he walked.

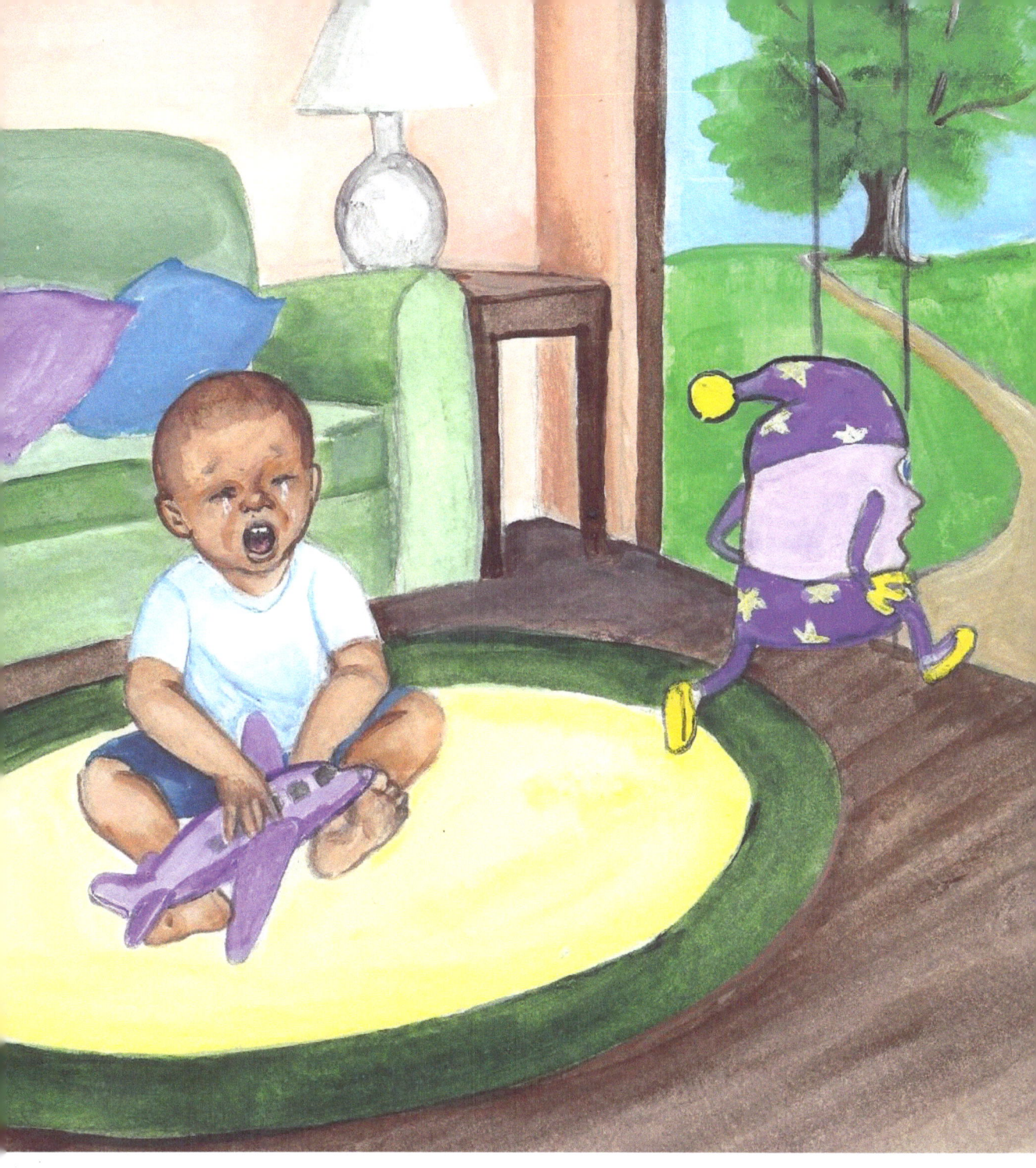

Oftentimes he tried sneaking up on Jacquay to help him get some rest. But Jacquay screamed and howled so loud he ran poor Mr. Sleep away.

Mr. Sleep only wanted to be Jacquay's friend.

He wanted Jacquay to be his friend too. Jacquay would be a great friend for Mr. Sleep.

But he did not understand that Mr. Sleep never wanted to harm him. So, he did not want to go to Mr. Sleep.

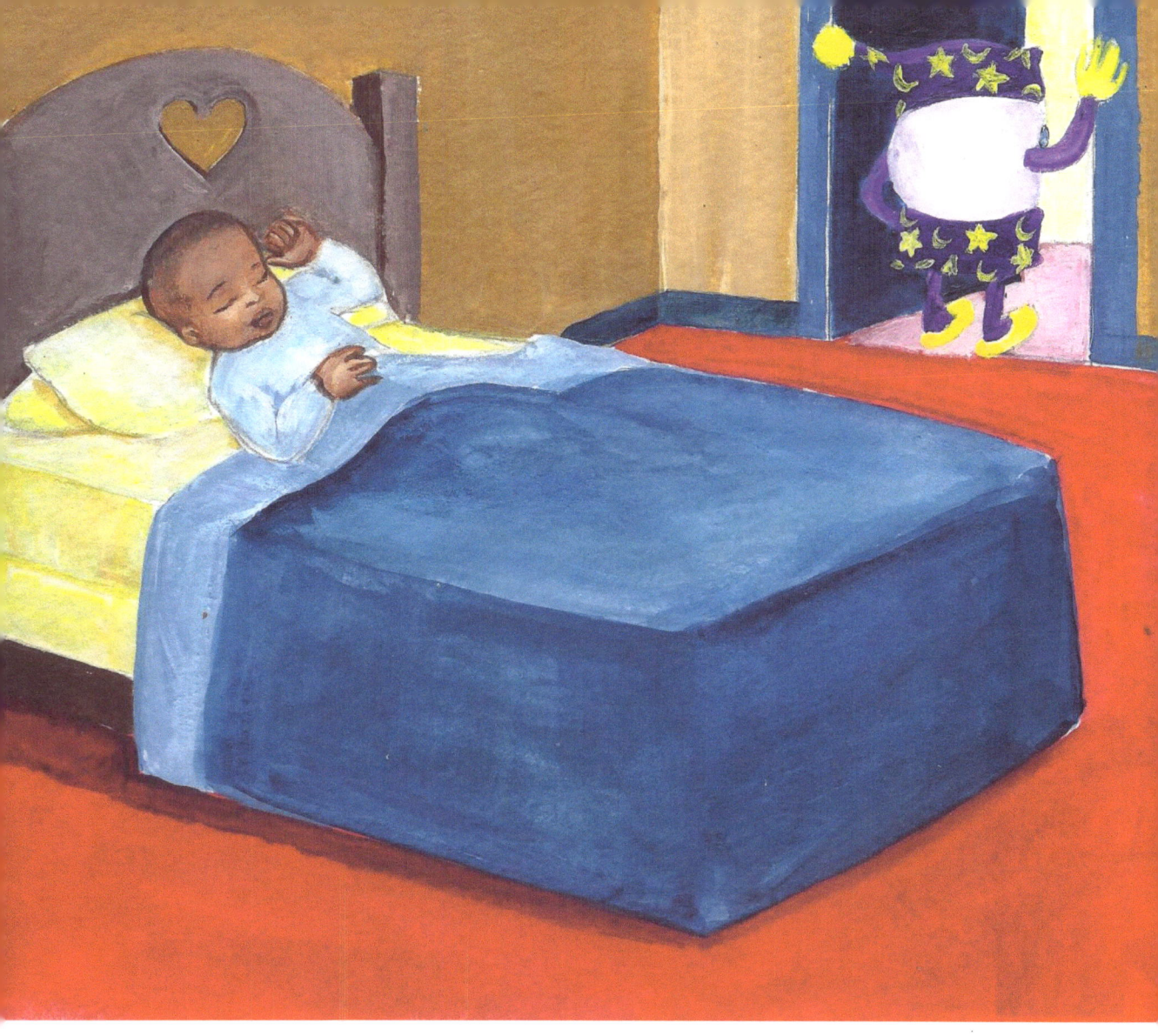

Only at night when it was quiet could Mr. Sleep sneak
upon Jacquay and put him to sleep. Then he took him
and held him in his warm cuddly arms, and made sure
he would grow healthy and strong. Early the next
morning he gave Jacquay a kiss and went away.

Jacquay woke, said his prayers,
took his shower, brushed his teeth,
combed his hair, ate breakfast, did
his chores.

AND WOW!

HIS FUN COULD THEN BEGIN!

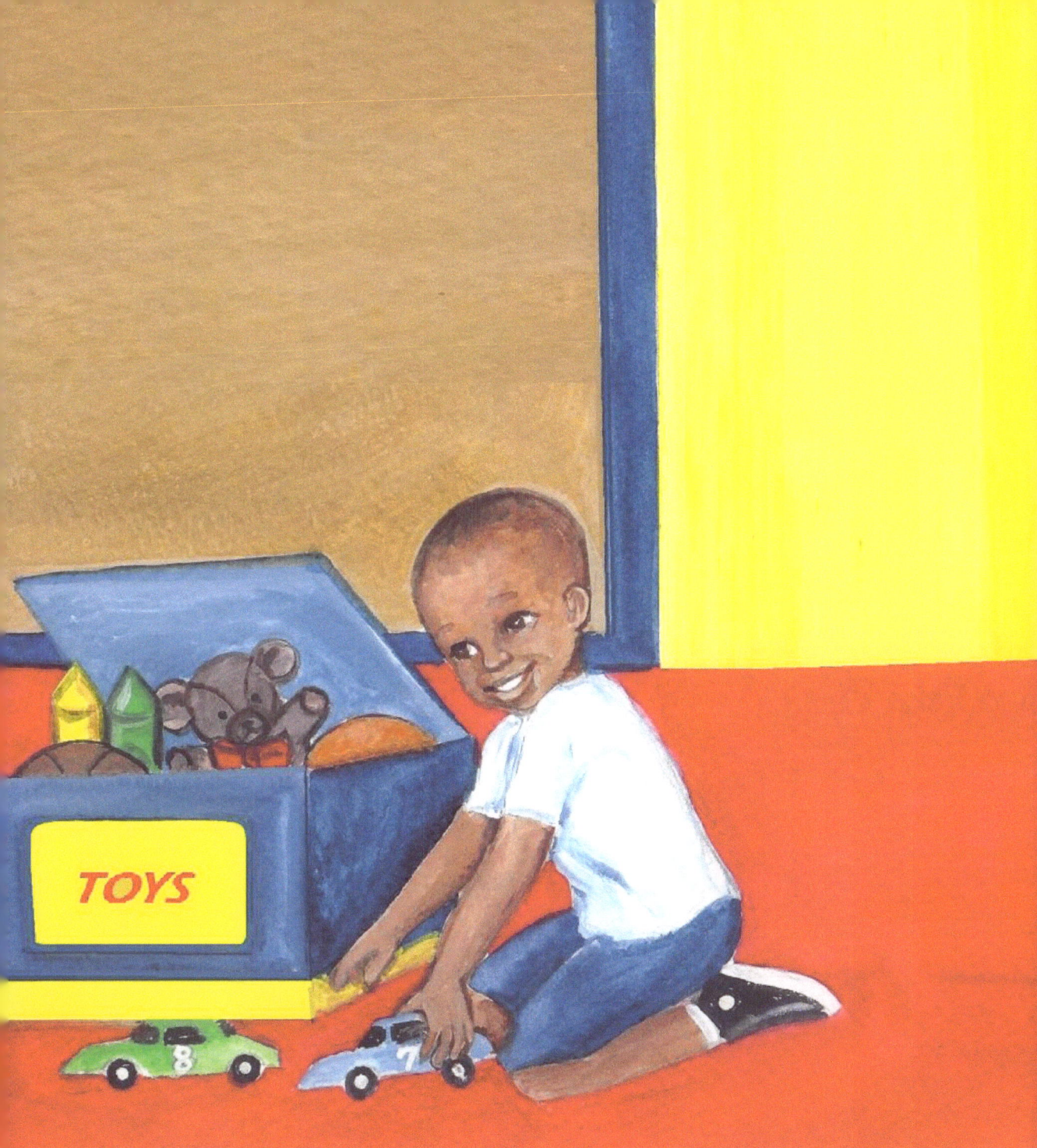

He would play with his toy racing cars, pushing them across the floors. Zoom! Zoom! Zoom! He played outdoors and indoors, and all across the floors.

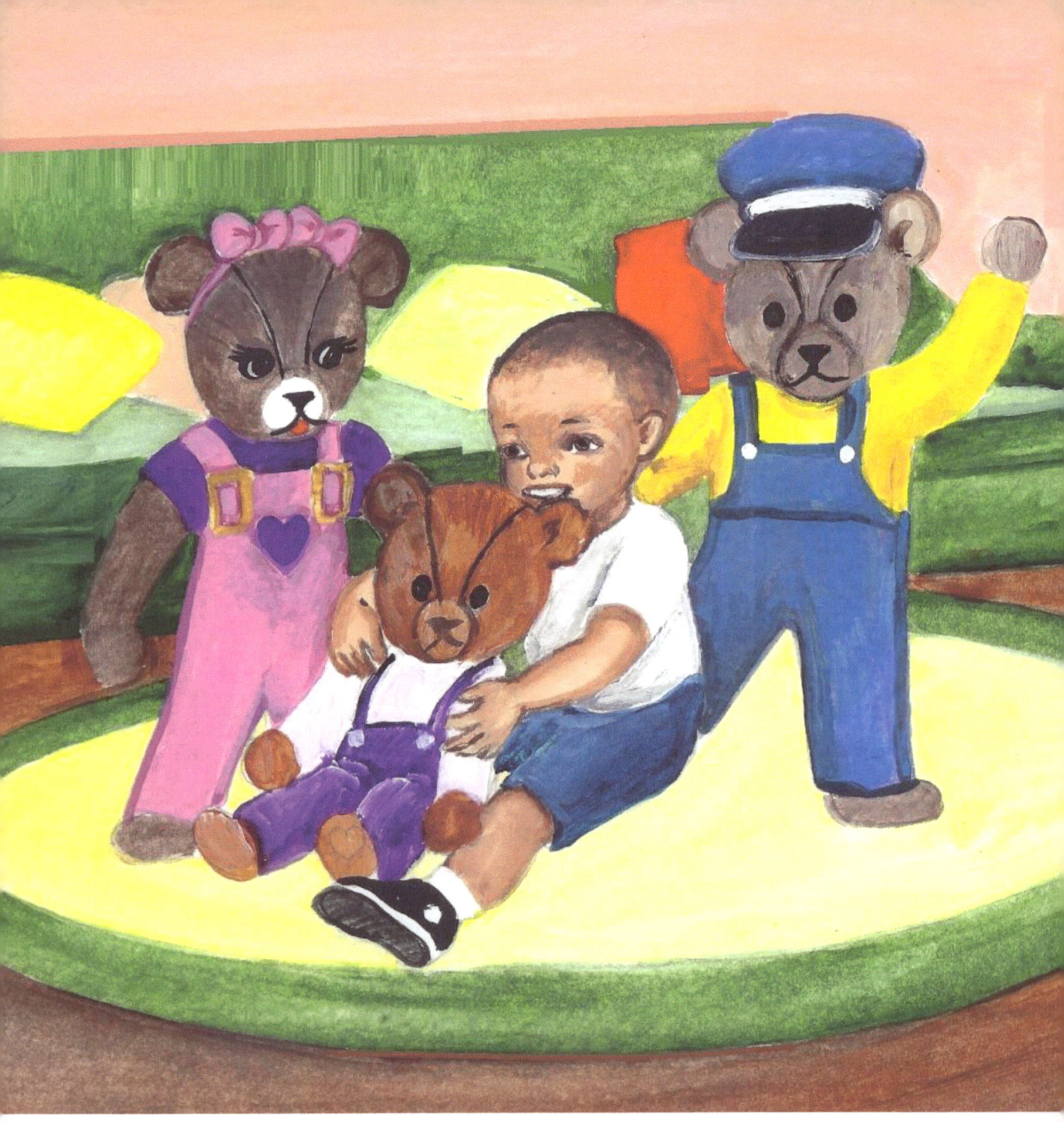

He played with big toys and little toys, short toys and long toys. He played on his bicycle and ate popsicles and fudgesicles. He played upstairs and downstairs with fun things like teddy bears.

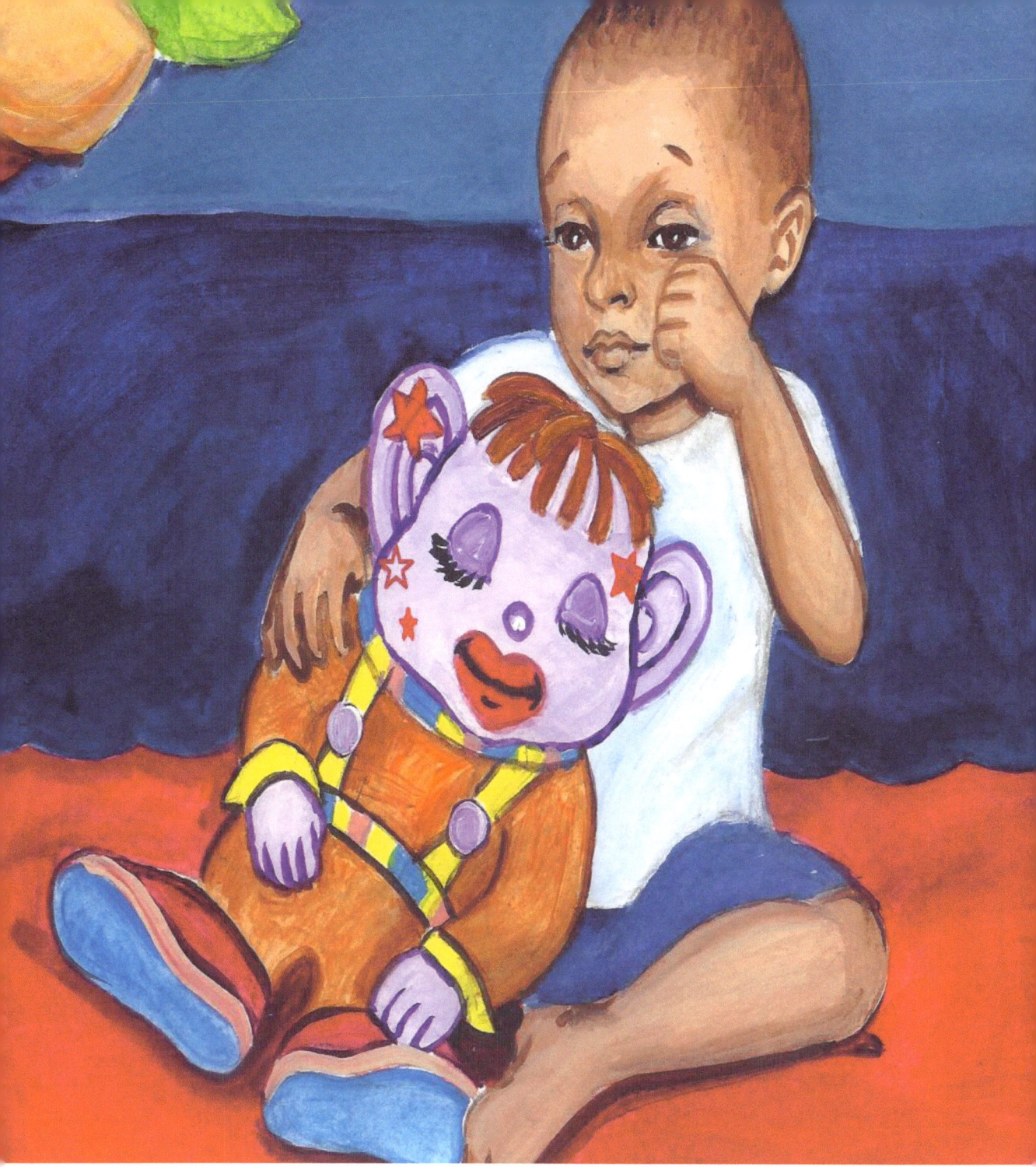

He ran up and down and bounced around. He played
with toy animals, and with Star, his friendly toy clown.

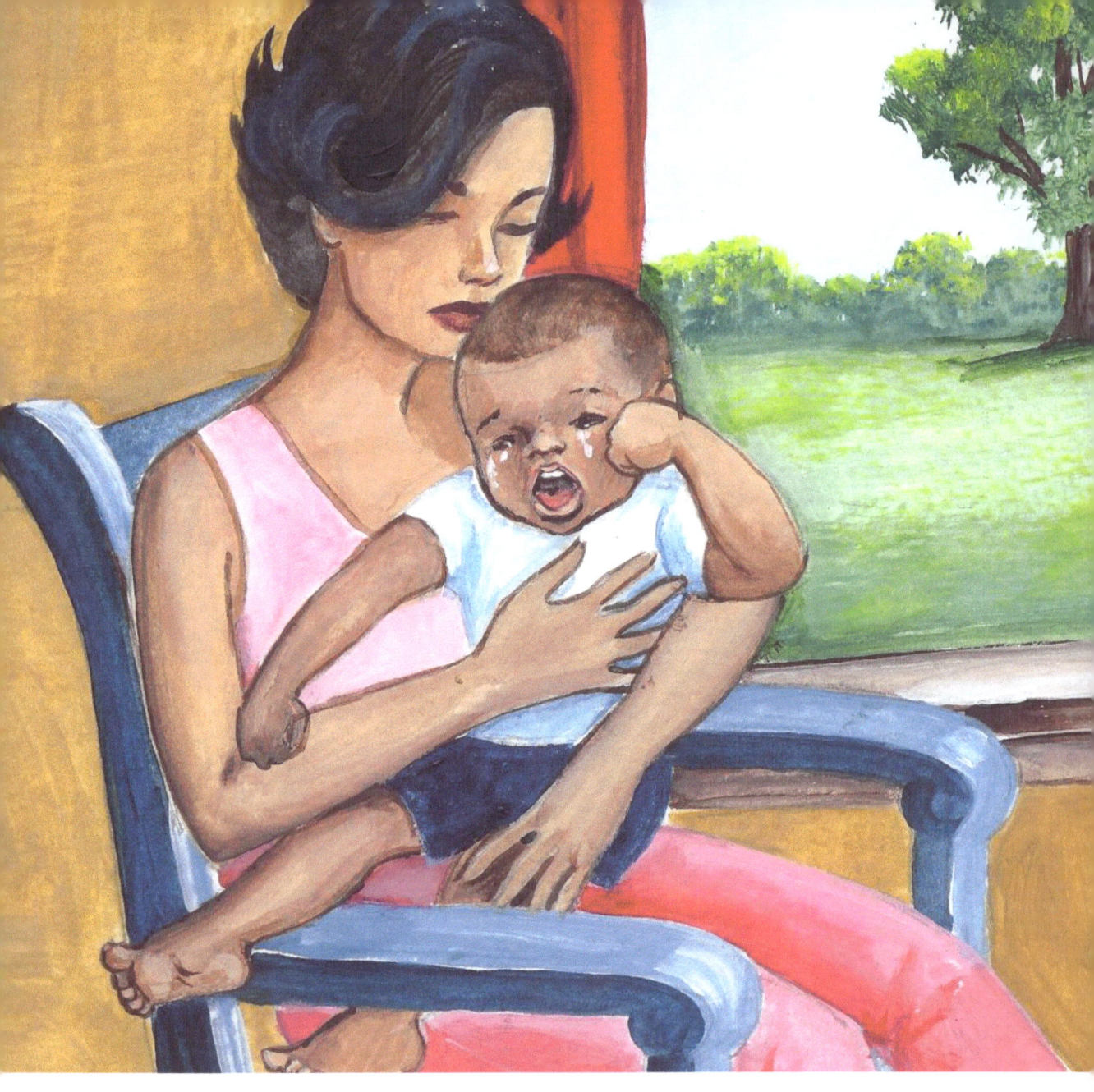

Jacquay played with every toy he had in his toy box. He then became tired and sleepy after playing for so long. But he pushed poor Mr. Sleep away and played some more. When his Mom placed him in her lap, he kicked and howled he would not take a nap.

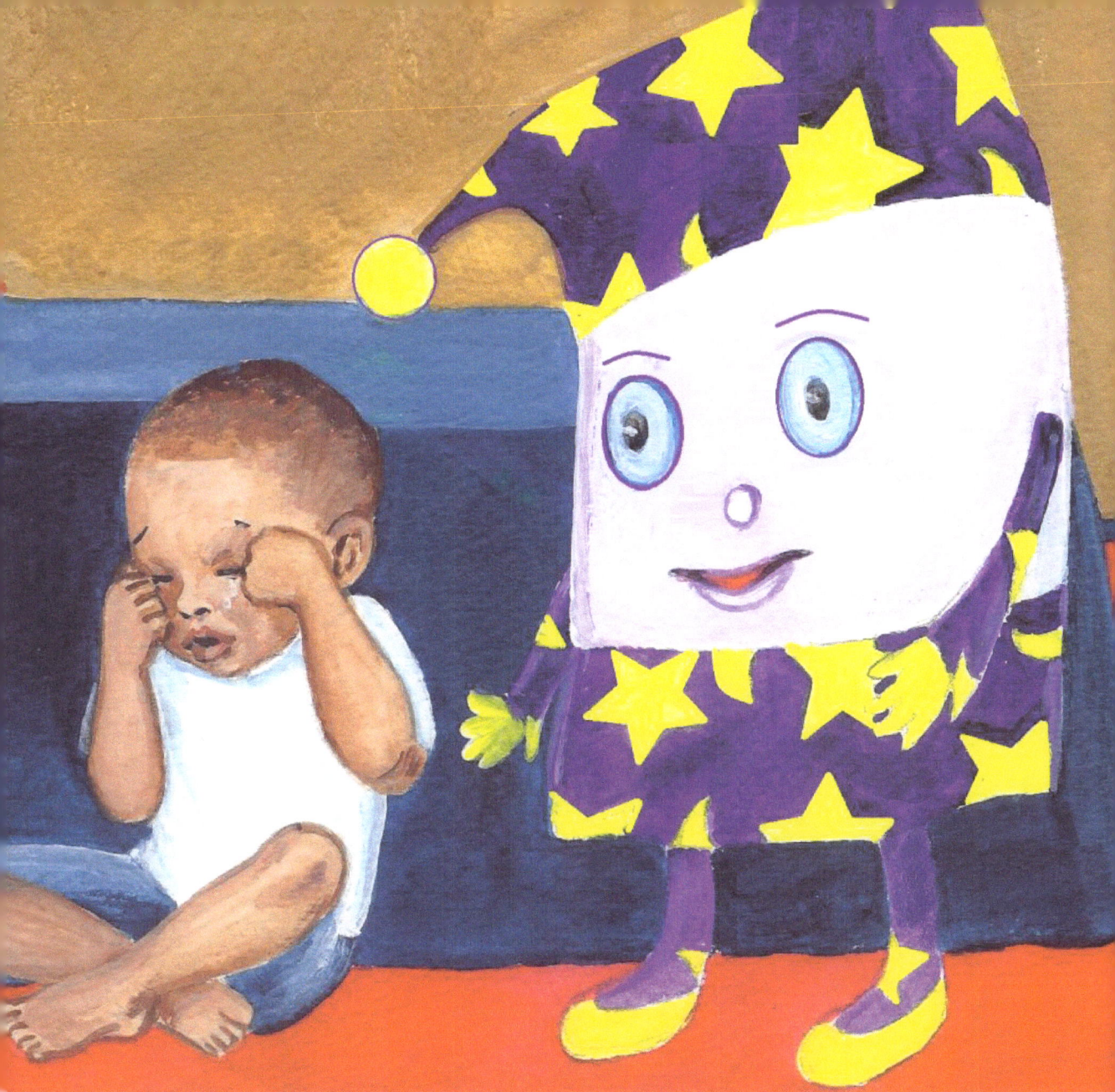

Jacquay was tired but he cried because he did not want to
go to sleep. Mr. Sleep came to him. "Don't cry Jacquay,"
said Mr. Sleep. "I'm not going to hurt you," Mr. Sleep
told him in a warm and friendly voice. "My name is Mr.
Sleep. You can call me Sleep. I only want to be your
friend. I can make you healthy. I can make you happy." *19*

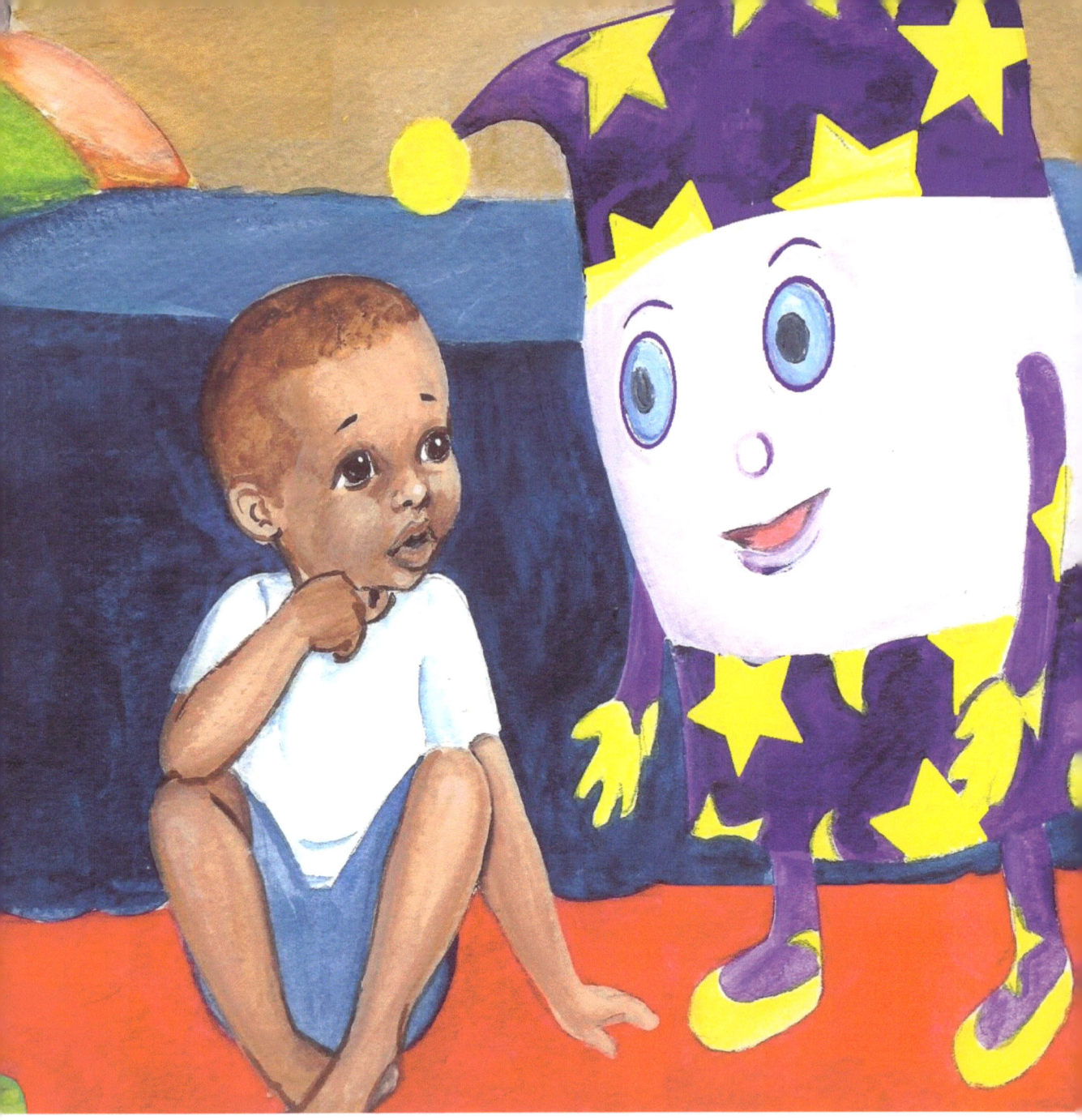

"You can make me healthy? You can make me
happy?" asked Jacquay. "How? How can you make
me happy? How can you make me healthy? I'm sad!
I'm angry! I don't want to go to sleep!"

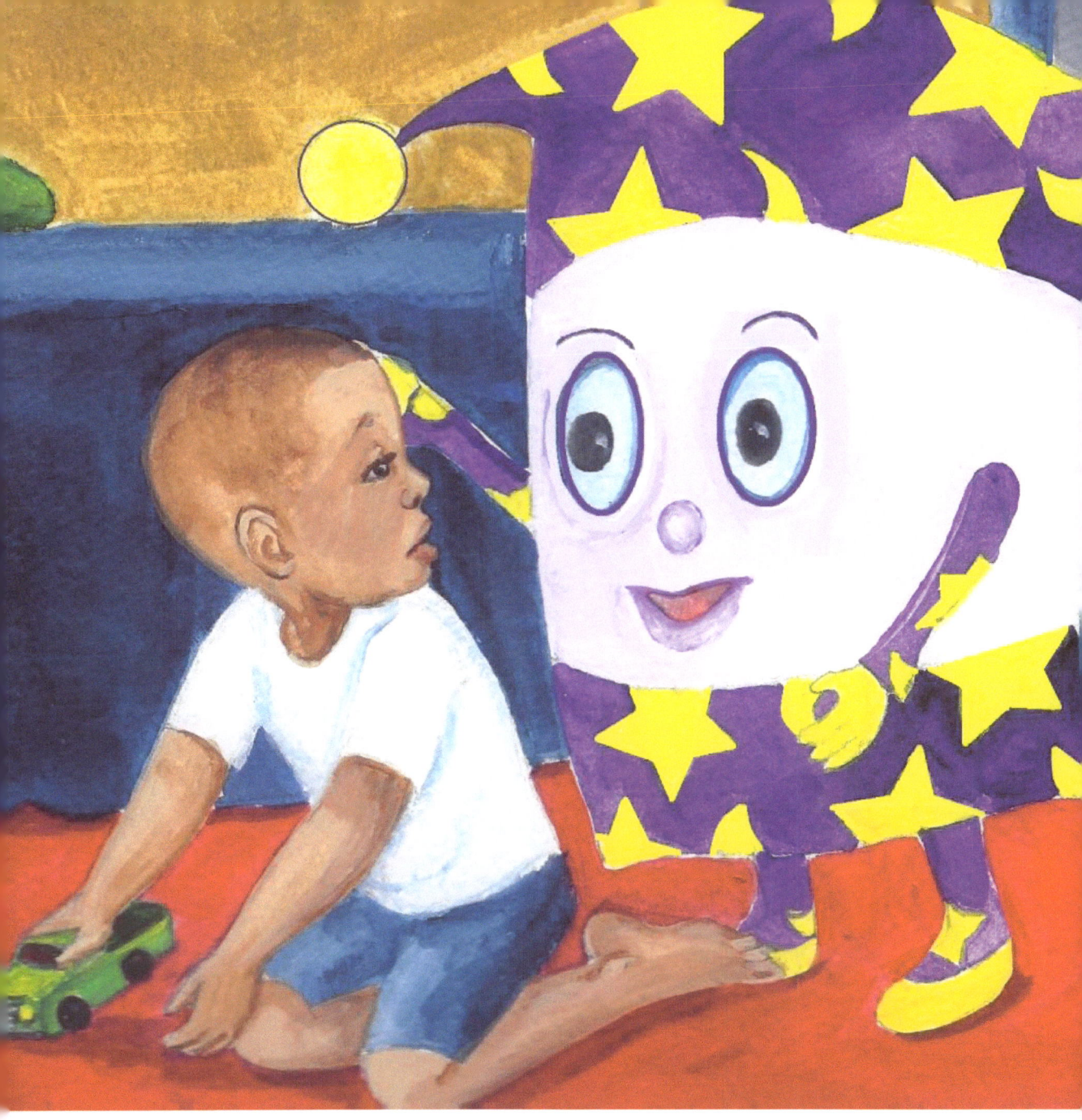

Mr. Sleep smiled, rubbed Jacquay on the head and said, "Now you are tired. When you go to sleep, I will make sure that you grow healthy and strong. You will wake up and not be tired anymore. You will be able to do all the things you like to do."

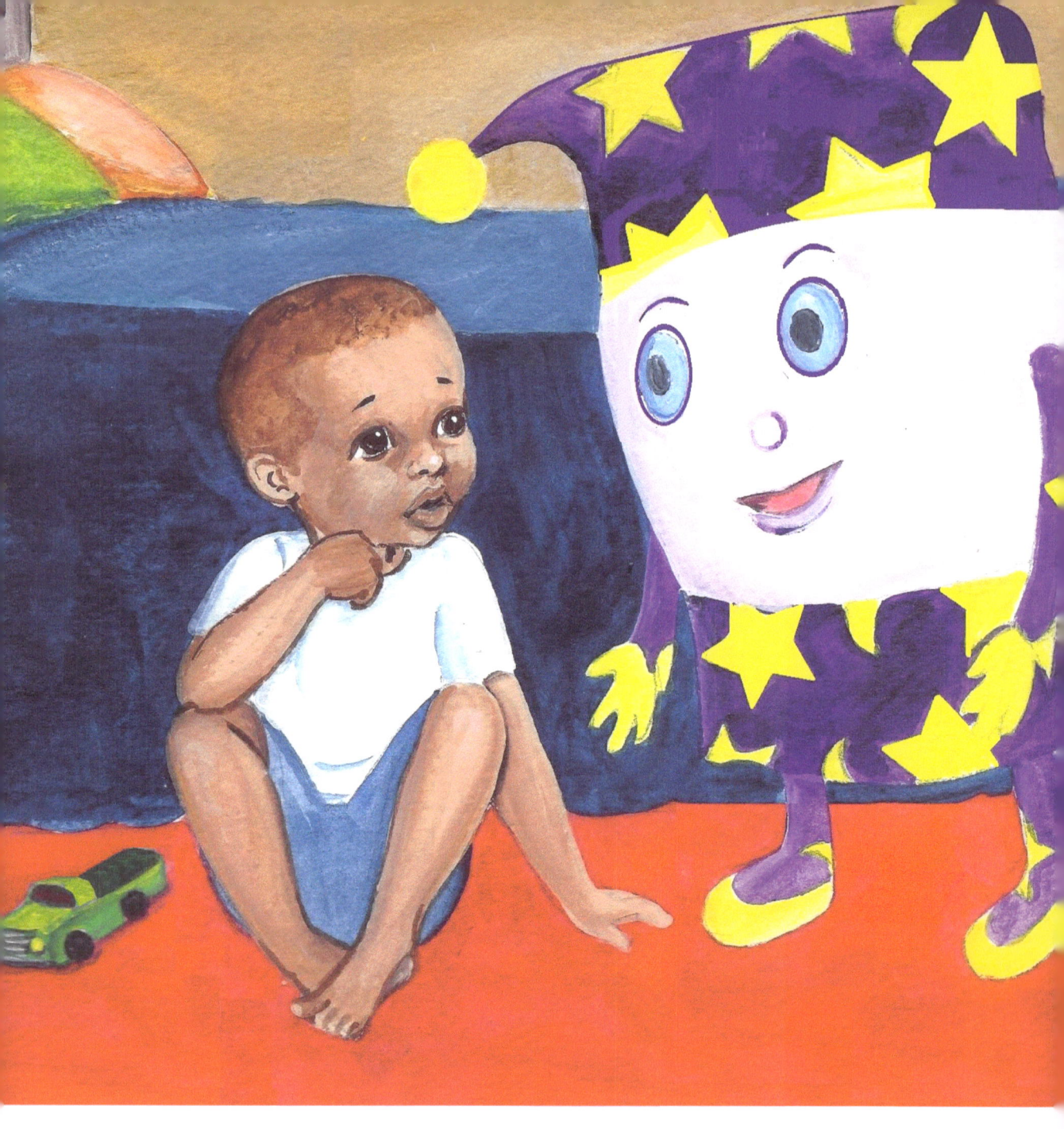

"You can run and play.

You can jump up and say,
WOW, IT'S A GREAT DAY!"

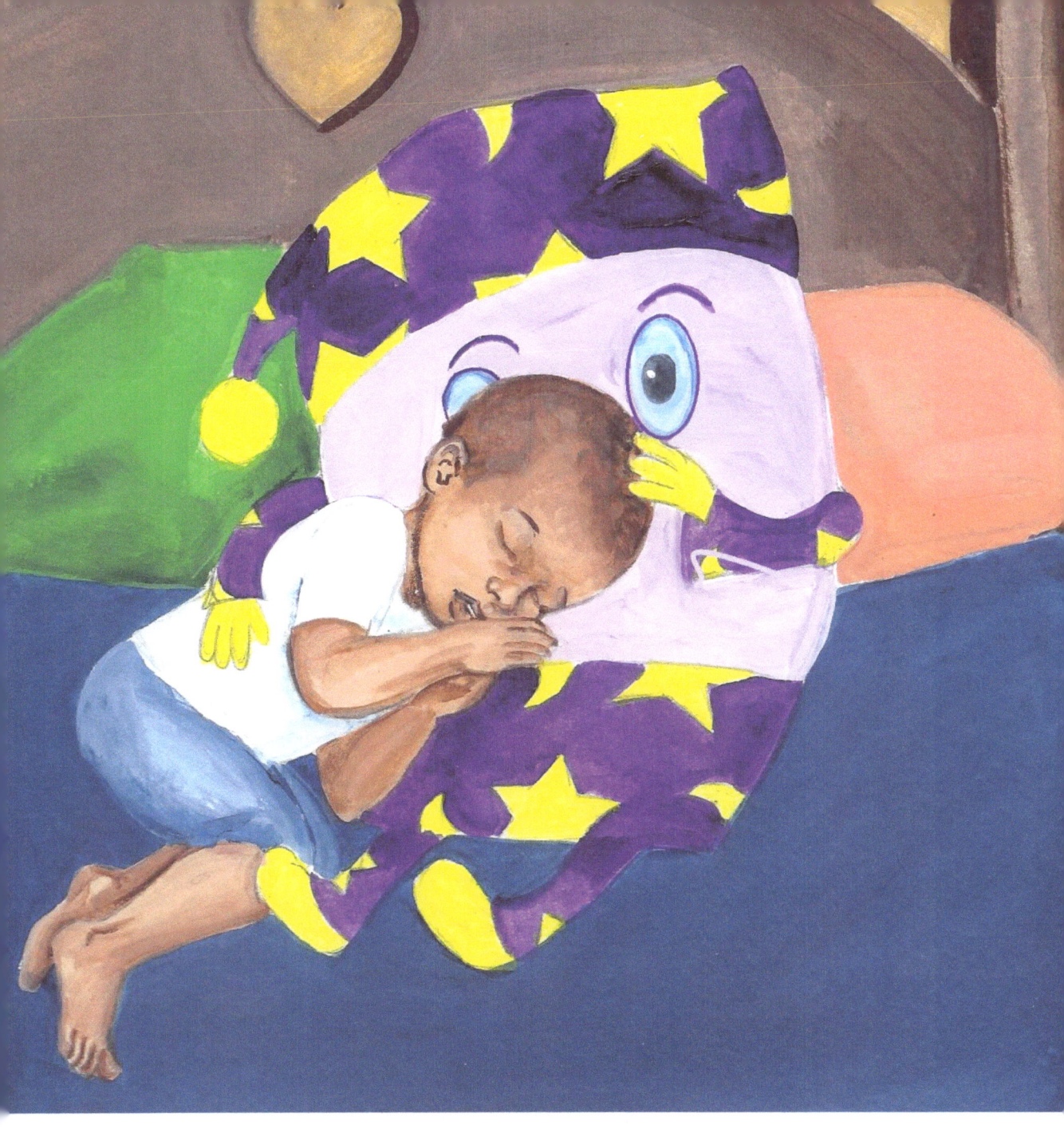

Jacquay looked at Mr. Sleep with a great big smile
on his face, and said, "GEE, MR. SLEEP, YOU'RE
A GREAT FRIEND!" He gave Mr. Sleep a great
big hug, fell in his arms and went to sleep.